Paleo Diet Recipes for every meal

Your guide to bring well-being and flavour to your table

Helena Stout

TABLE OF CONTENTS

Readers acknowledge that the author is not engaging in the rendering of legal, financial, medical or professional advice. The content within this book has been derived from various sources. Please consult a licensed professional before attempting any techniques outlined in this book. By reading this document, the reader agrees that under no circumstances is the author responsible for any losses, 5 direct or indirect, which are incurred as a result of the use of information contained within this document, including, but not limited to, — errors, omissions, or inaccuracies.

BREAKFAST

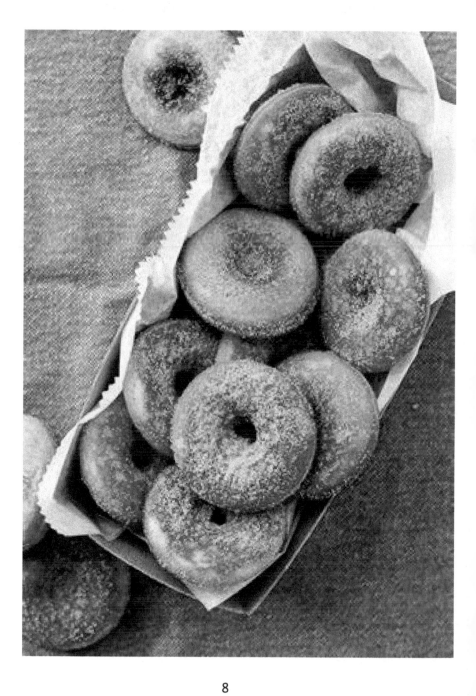

Pancetta Baked Eggs

Prep time: 15 minutes

Cooking time: 15 minutes

Servings: 2

Ingredients:

- 2 eggs

- 1 teaspoon coconut oil

- 2 pancetta slices

- ¼ teaspoon ground black pepper

Directions:
1. Brush the ramekins with coconut oil.
2. Put pancetta slices in the ramekins.
3. Then crack the eggs above the pancetta.
4. Sprinkle the eggs with ground black pepper and cover with the foil.
5. Pierce the foil with the help of the toothpicks.
6. Preheat the oven to 365F.
7. Put the ramekins with eggs in the oven and cook them for 15 minutes.
8. Then remove the foil from the ramekins and let the eggs rest for 5 minutes.

Nutrition value/serving:

Calories 186, fat 14.6, fiber 0.1, carbs 0.8, protein 12.6

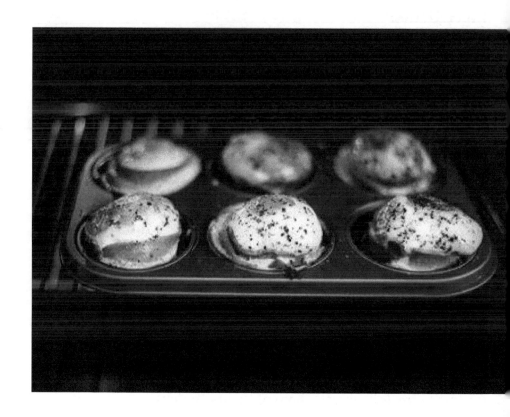

Morning Egg Salad

Prep time: 10 minutes

Cooking time: 0 minutes

Servings: 6

Ingredients:
- ½ cup of coconut yogurt
- 4 eggs, hard-boiled
- ½ cup celery stalk, chopped
- 1 tablespoon chives, chopped
- 1 teaspoon chili flakes
- ½ red onion, chopped
- 2 oz pickles, chopped
- ½ teaspoon salt
- 1 tablespoon fresh dill, chopped

Directions:
1. Peel the eggs and chop them.
2. Put the chopped eggs in the salad bowl and add celery stalk, chives, chili flakes, red onion, and pickles.

3. After this, in the separated bowl mix up coconut yogurt, salt, and fresh dill. Whisk the mixture gently.
4. Pour the yogurt mixture over the salad. Mix up the salad well.

Nutrition value/serving:

Calories 59, fat 3.3, fiber 0.5, carbs 3, protein 4.3

Chicken Salad with Tahini

Prep time: 15 minutes

Cooking time: 20 minutes

Servings: 4

Ingredients:
- 1 tablespoon tahini sauce
- 1 teaspoon sesame seeds
- 1-pound chicken breast, skinless, boneless
- 1 cup lettuce, chopped
- ½ teaspoon salt
- 1 teaspoon olive oil
- 1 teaspoon ground black pepper
- 1 tablespoon coconut cream

Directions:
1. Chop the chicken breast and mix it up with olive oil, salt, and ground black pepper.
2. Put the chicken in the skillet and flatten it in one layer.
3. Cook the chicken in the preheated to 365F for 20 minutes.
4. Meanwhile, put the chopped lettuce in the salad bowl.

5. Add sesame seeds, salt, and coconut cream.

6. Then add cooked chicken and mix up the salad.

7. Sprinkle the salad with tahini sauce.

Nutrition value/serving:

calories 167, fat 6.3, fiber 0.5, carbs 1.4, protein 24.6

Egg with Bacon

Prep time: 10 minutes

Cooking time: 17 minutes

Servings: 2

Ingredients:

- 1 teaspoon chives, chopped

- ¼ teaspoon minced garlic

- 2 teaspoons coconut cream

- 2 bacon slices

- 2 eggs, beaten

- 1 teaspoon coconut oil

Directions:

1. Put the coconut oil in the skillet and melt it up on the medium heat.
2. Then place the bacon in the hot oil and cook it for 1 minute from each side.
3. Meanwhile, in the mixing bowl mix up chives, minced garlic, coconut cream, and eggs.
4. Pour the egg mixture over the bacon and close the lid.
5. Cook the meal for 15 minutes over the medium-low heat.

Nutrition value/serving: calories 197, fat 15.8, fiber 0.1, carbs 1, protein 12.7

Cinnamon Donuts

Prep time: 20 minutes

Cooking time: 25 minute

Servings: 4

Ingredients:
- 4 tablespoons almond flour
- ½ teaspoon baking soda
- 1 teaspoon lemon juice
- 1 teaspoon ground cinnamon
- 1 egg, beaten
- 1 teaspoon vanilla extract
- 1 tablespoon Erythritol
- 1 tablespoon coconut oil

Directions:
1. In the mixing bowl mix up almond flour, baking soda, lemon juice, ground cinnamon, egg, and vanilla extract.
2. Knead the soft and non-sticky dough.
3. Then roll up the dough.
4. Make the donuts with the help of the cutter.

5. Line the baking tray with baking paper.

6. Then brush it with coconut oil.

7. Put the donuts in the tray.

8. Cook them for 25 minutes at 365F.

9. When the donuts are cooked, sprinkle them with Erythritol.

Nutrition value/serving:

calories 210, fat 18.5, fiber 3.3, carbs 6.7, protein 7.4

Chili Breakfast Balls

Prep time: 10 minutes

Cooking time: 6 minutes

Servings: 2

Ingredients:

- 7 oz ground beef

- 1 chili, chopped

- ½ teaspoon chili flakes

- ¼ teaspoon salt

- 1 egg, beaten

- ½ teaspoon dried parsley

- ¼ teaspoon ground nutmeg

- 1 teaspoon coconut oil

Directions:

1. In the mixing bowl mix up ground beef, chili, chili flakes, salt, egg, dried parsley, and ground nutmeg.
2. Make the small meatballs.
3. Melt the coconut oil in the skillet.

4. Put the meatballs in the hot coconut oil in one layer and cook them for 3 minutes from each side over the medium heat.

5. Dry the cooked meatballs with the help of the paper towel, if needed.

Nutrition value/serving:

calories 236, fat 10.6, fiber 0.1, carbs 0.4, protein 32.9

LUNCH

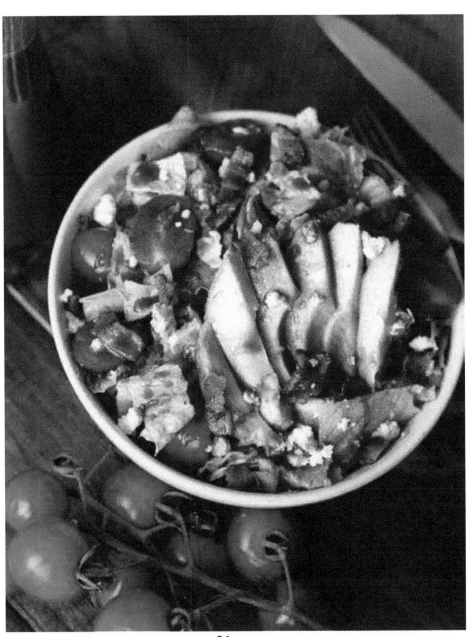

Cuban Sandwich

Prep time: 15 minutes

Cooking time: 20 minutes

Servings: 2

Ingredients:

- 1 plantain, peeled

- 1 egg, whisked

- 1 teaspoon flax meal

- ½ teaspoon salt

- 2 pork chops, chopped

- 1 teaspoon ground black pepper

- 2 ham slices

- ½ teaspoon chili pepper

- 1 teaspoon coconut oil

Directions:

1. Sprinkle the pork chops with ground black pepper and chili pepper.
2. Then heat up the coconut oil in the skillet.

3. Put the pork chops in the hot coconut oil and cook for 5 minutes form each side or until they are cooked.
4. Meanwhile, slice the plantain on 4 horizontal slices.
5. When the pork chops are cooked, transfer them on the plate.
6. Pour the whisked egg in the skillet and fry it for 3 minutes.
7. Then transfer the egg on the chopping board and cut into halves.
8. Put the sliced plantain in the skillet and fry it for 1 minute from each side.
9. Then put 2 plantain slices in the plate and top them with pork chops.
10. Then add the fried egg halves, salt, flax meal, and ham slices.
11. Top the sandwich with remaining plantain slices.

Nutrition value/serving:

calories 472, fat 27.6, fiber 3.2, carbs 31.3, protein 27

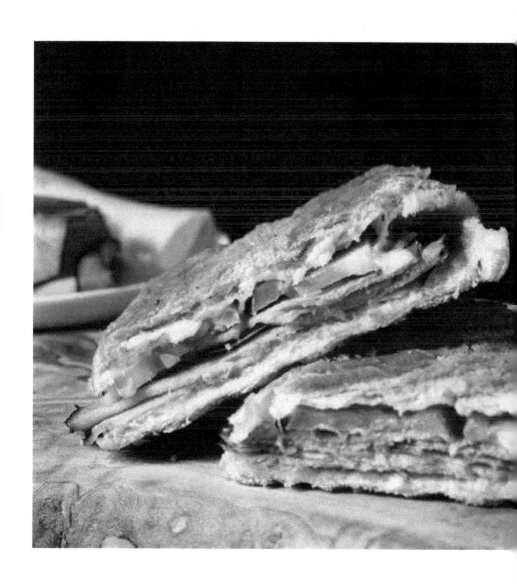

BLT Salad

Prep time: 10 minutes

Cooking time: 7 minutes

Servings: 3

Ingredients:

- 1 ½ cup lettuce, chopped

- 1-pound chicken breast, skinless, boneless

- 1 cup grape tomatoes

- 3 bacon slices, chopped, cooked

- 1 teaspoon coconut oil

- ½ teaspoon salt

- ½ teaspoon white pepper

- ¼ cup of coconut yogurt

- 1 teaspoon apple cider vinegar

Directions:

1. Chop the chicken breast on the small cubes and sprinkle them with salt and white pepper.
2. Add coconut oil and mix up the chicken well.

3. Put it in the skillet and cook for 7 minutes over the medium heat. Stir the chicken with the help of the spatula from time to time.
4. After this, transfer the cooked chicken in the salad bowl.
5. Add chopped lettuce, cooked bacon, and coconut yogurt.
6. Cut the grape tomatoes on the halves and add them in the salad.
7. Sprinkle it with apple cider vinegar and shake well.

Nutrition value/serving:

calories 313, fat 13.7, fiber 1, carbs 4.8, protein 40.1

Jar Taco Salad

Prep time: 10 minutes

Cooking time: 10 minutes

Servings: 4

Ingredients:

- 1-pound ground beef

- 1 teaspoon coconut oil

- 1 teaspoon taco seasonings

- 1 onion, diced

- 1 teaspoon salt

- 1 cup Romaine lettuce, chopped

- 1 avocado, chopped

- 1 teaspoon minced garlic

- 2 teaspoons lemon juice

- 4 tomatoes, chopped

- 1 tablespoon olive oil

- ½ teaspoon dried cilantro

Directions:

1. In the mixing bowl mix up ground beef and taco seasoning.
2. Then transfer the meat mixture in the skillet, add coconut oil, and diced onion.
3. Close the lid and cook the ingredients for 5 minutes.
4. Then open the lid and mix it up.
5. Cook the ingredients for 5 minutes more.
6. After this, transfer the cooked ground mixture in the mason jars.
7. Add salt and the layer of Romaine lettuce.
8. Then add the layer of the avocado, minced garlic, and tomatoes.
9. In the shallow bowl mix yo dried cilantro, olive oil, and lemon juice.
10. Sprinkle every salad serving with lemon juice dressing. Close the mason jars and store them in the fridge for up to 2 hours.

Nutrition value/serving:

calories 392, fat 21.8, fiber 5.6, carbs 12.9, protein 36.9

Ham Chowder

Prep time: 10 minutes

Cooking time: 30 minutes

Servings: 4

Ingredients:

- 7 oz ham, chopped

- 3 celery stalks, chopped

- ½ green onion, chopped

- ¼ teaspoon garlic powder

- ½ carrot, grated

- ½ cup turnip, chopped

- 3 cups chicken stock

- 1 teaspoon coconut oil

- 1 teaspoon salt

- ½ teaspoon dried rosemary

- 1/3 teaspoon chili flakes

Directions:

1. Put the coconut oil in the saucepan and melt it.
2. Then add grated carrot and green onion.
3. Roast the vegetables for 5 minutes. Stir them from time to time to avoid burning.
4. Then add celery stalk, turnip, garlic powder, salt, rosemary, and chili flakes. Stir the ingredients well and add chicken stock.
5. Bring the mixture to boil and simmer for 10 minutes.
6. Then add chopped ham and cook the soup for 15 minutes more.

Nutrition value/serving:

calories 109, fat 5.9, fiber 1.5, carbs 5, protein 9.1

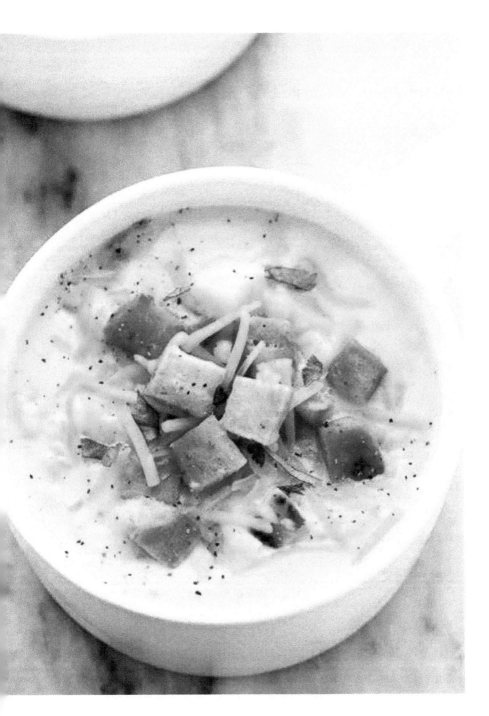

Bison Stew

Prep time: 20 minutes

Cooking time: 25 minutes

Servings: 4

Ingredients:

- 1-pound ground bison

- 3 oz rutabaga, chopped

- ½ cup kale, chopped

- 2 cups vegetable stock

- ½ cup Brussel sprouts, roughly chopped

- 1 teaspoon smoked paprika

- ½ teaspoon salt

- ½ teaspoon ground cumin

- ¼ teaspoon dried thyme

- 1 teaspoon cayenne pepper

Directions:

1. In the mixing bowl mix up ground bison, smoked paprika, salt, ground cumin, dried thyme, and cayenne pepper.

2. Then put the meat mixture in the pan.
3. Add vegetable stock and bring the mixture to boil. Cook it for 5 minutes more.
4. After this, add rutabaga, Brussel sprouts, and simmer the stew for 10 minutes over the medium heat.
5. When the Brussel sprouts are soft, add kale and cook the stew for 10 minutes on the low heat.
6. Let the cooked stew rest for 20 minutes.

Nutrition value/serving:

calories 294, fat 17.5, fiber 1.7, carbs 4.8, protein 28.2

Crab Stew

Prep time: 10 minutes

Cooking time: 15 minutes

Servings: 3

Ingredients:

- 14 oz crab meat, chopped

- 2 shallots, chopped

- 1 jalapeno pepper, sliced

- 1 tomato, chopped

- ¼ cup tomato juice

- 1 teaspoon cumin seeds

- ¼ teaspoon fennel seeds

- 1 cup fish stock

Directions:

1. Put shallots in the saucepan.
2. Add jalapeno pepper, cumin seeds, fennel seeds, and fish stock.
3. Add tomato and tomato juice.

4. Bring the mixture to boil and simmer it for 5 minutes.

5. Then add chopped crab meat and cook the stew on the low heat for 10 minutes.

6. Let the cooked stew rest for 10 minutes before serving.

Nutrition value/serving:

calories 144, fat 3.3, fiber 0.6, carbs 4.9, protein 18.9

Veg & Meat Stew

Prep time: 10 minutes

Cooking time: 55 minutes

Servings: 2

Ingredients:

- 4 oz asparagus, chopped

- 4 oz broccoli, chopped

- 10 oz beef shank, chopped

- 1 cup chicken stock

- ½ teaspoon peppercorn

- 1 bay leaf

- 1 teaspoon salt

- 1 teaspoon tapioca flour

Directions:

1. Pour the chicken stock in the pan.
2. Add beef shank, peppercorns, bay leaf, and salt.
3. Then close the lid and cook the meat mixture for 40 minutes on the medium heat.

4. After this, add asparagus and broccoli.

5. Cook the stew for 10 minutes more.

6. Add tapioca flour and stir the stew until flour is dissolved.

7. Cook the stew for 5 minutes more. All the ingredients of the stew should be very soft.

Nutrition value/serving:

calories 328, fat 9.6, fiber 2.9, carbs 8.1, protein 51

SIDE DISHES

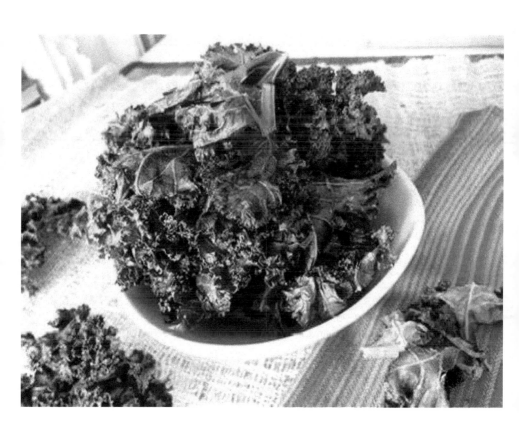

Spaghetti Squash Pasta

Prep time: 15 minutes

Cooking time: 40 minutes

Servings: 3

Ingredients:

- 8 oz spaghetti squash, halved, deseeded

- 1 tablespoon coconut cream

- 1 teaspoon cassava flour

- 1 tablespoon sunflower oil

- 1 teaspoon coconut oil

- ½ teaspoon salt

Directions:

1. Sprinkle the spaghetti squash in the oven and bake it at 365F for 30 minutes.
2. Then cool it little and shred with the help of the fork.
3. Transfer the shredded squash in the skillet and add the sunflower oil.
4. Cook the ingredients for 3 minutes.
5. Then add cassava flour, coconut cream, and salt. Stir the mixture until homogenous and close the lid.
6. Cook the pasta for 5 minutes on the low heat.

Nutrition value/serving:

calories 129, fat 7.8, fiber 0.4, carbs 14.8, protein 0.6

Zucchini Fettuccine

Prep time: 10 minutes

Cooking time: 7 minutes

Servings: 4

Ingredients:

- 2 large zucchinis, trimmed

- ¼ cup organic almond milk

- ½ teaspoon ground black pepper

- 1 teaspoon coconut oil

Directions:

1. Toss the coconut oil in the pan and melt it.
2. Then add almond milk and ground black pepper.
3. Bring the liquid to boil on the low heat.
4. Meanwhile, make the zucchini fettuccine with the help of the potato peeler.
5. Put the fettuccine in the hot almond milk and stir well.
6. Cook the meal for 2 minutes on the medium heat.

Nutrition value/serving:

calories 40, fat 1.6, fiber 1.9, carbs 6.1, protein 2

Kelp Noodles

Prep time: 10 minutes

Cooking time: 20 minutes

Servings: 4

Ingredients:

- 1 package kelp noodles

- 1 tablespoon coconut cream

- ½ teaspoon salt

- 1 cup of water

Directions:

1. Preheat the water until warm and put the kelp noodles inside.
2. Let the noodles for 20 minutes.
3. Then remove them from the water and sprinkle with salt and coconut cream.
4. Stir the noodles gently.

Nutrition value/serving:

calories 10, fat 0.9, fiber 0.3, carbs 0.5, protein 0.1

Eggplant Lasagna

Prep time: 10 minutes

Cooking time: 10 minutes

Servings: 4

Ingredients:
- ½ teaspoon ground paprika

- ½ teaspoon ground turmeric

- 1 teaspoon ground cumin

- ½ teaspoon salt

- 1 tablespoon coconut oil, melted

- 2 large eggplants

Directions:
1. Slice the eggplants on the horizontal slices.
2. Rub every eggplant slice with paprika, turmeric, cumin, and salt.
3. Then sprinkle them with coconut oil.
4. Preheat the grill to 375F.
5. Place the eggplant slices in the grill in one layer and cook them for 2 minutes from each side.

Nutrition value/serving:

calories 102, fat 4.1, fiber 9.9, carbs 16.7, protein 2.8

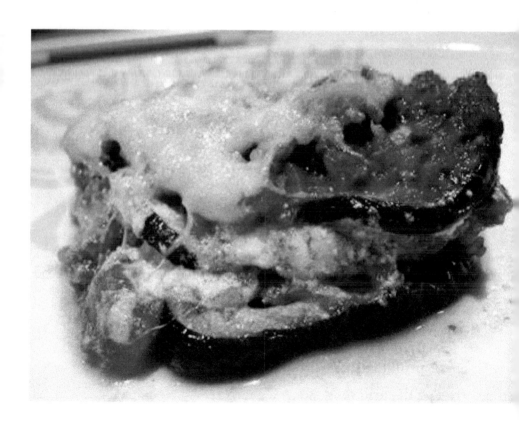

Vegetable Medley

Prep time: 10 minutes

Cooking time: 30 minutes

Servings: 2

Ingredients:
- ½ cup cauliflower, chopped

- 1 cup radish, chopped

- ½ cup white mushrooms, chopped

- 1 teaspoon dried thyme

- 1 teaspoon salt

- 1 tablespoon lemon juice

- 4 oz beef broth

- 1 tablespoon sesame oil

- ½ teaspoon ground black pepper

Directions:
1. In the mixing bowl mix up chopped cauliflower, radish, mushrooms, dried thyme, salt, lemon juice, sesame oil, and ground black pepper.

2. Put the vegetables in the saucepan, add beef broth, and sesame oil.

3. Close the lid and cook the vegetable medley for 30 minutes on the medium heat.

Nutrition value/serving:

calories 93, fat 7.4, fiber 2.1, carbs 4.9, protein 2.8

Italian Style Kale

Prep time: 15 minutes

Cooking time: 9 minutes

Servings: 4

Ingredients:

- 1 tablespoon coconut oil

- 3 cups kale, chopped

- 1 teaspoon salt

- 1 cup chicken stock

- 1 teaspoon Italian seasonings

Directions:

1. Pour the chicken stock in the saucepan and bring to boil.
2. Add kale and cook it for 4 minutes.
3. Then transfer the kale in the pan.
4. Add Italian seasonings, salt, and coconut oil.
5. Roast the kale for 5 minutes.

Nutrition value/serving:

calories 57, fat 3.5, fiber 0.8, carbs 5.4, protein 1.7

Grilled Yellow Squash

Prep time: 15 minutes

Cooking time: 6 minutes

Servings: 2

Ingredients:

- 8 oz yellow squash, deseeded

- 1 teaspoon olive oil

- 1 teaspoon white pepper

Directions:

1. Cut the yellow squash into the wedges and sprinkle with olive oil and white pepper.
2. Preheat the grill to 375F.
3. Put the yellow squash wedges in the grill in one layer.
4. Grill the vegetables for 3 minutes from each side.

Nutrition value/serving:

calories 41, fat 2.6, fiber 1.5, carbs 4.5, protein 1.5

SNACK

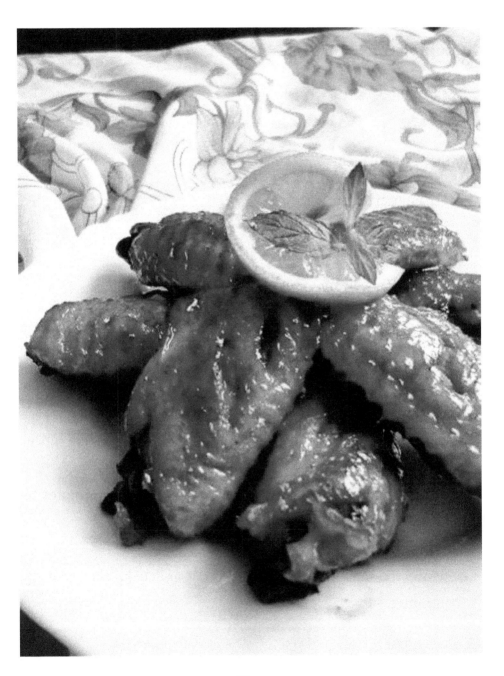

Lemon Chicken Wings

Prep time: 15 minutes

Cooking time: 25 minutes

Servings: 4

Ingredients:

- 4 chicken wings

- 1 teaspoon lemon zest, grated

- 1 tablespoon lemon juice

- 1 teaspoon avocado oil

- ½ teaspoon ground paprika

- ¼ teaspoon salt

Directions:

1. Sprinkle the chicken wings with lemon zest, lemon juice, avocado oil, paprika, and salt.
2. Mix up the chicken wings and leave them for 10 minutes to marinate.
3. After this, preheat the oven to 365F.
4. Place the chicken wings in the tray and bake them for 25 minutes.

Nutrition value/serving:

calories 28, fat 1.9, fiber 0.2, carbs 0.4, protein 2.4

Lamb Meatballs

Prep time: 20 minutes

Cooking time: 10 minutes

Servings: 6

Ingredients:

- 1-pound ground lamb

- 1 garlic clove, minced

- 1 teaspoon ground cumin

- 1 teaspoon minced onion

- 1 teaspoon salt

- 1 teaspoon coconut oil

Directions:

1. In the mixing bowl mix up ground lamb, minced garlic clove, cumin, minced onion, and salt.
2. After this, make the small meatballs from the lamb mixture.
3. Put the coconut oil in the skillet and heat it up.
4. When the coconut oil is hot, put the lamb meatballs in it and cook for 3 minutes from each side on the medium heat.

Nutrition value/serving:

calories 149, fat 6.4, fiber 0.1, carbs 0.4, protein 21.3

Turkey Meatballs with Chives

Prep time: 15 minutes

Cooking time: 25 minutes

Servings: 8

Ingredients:

- 16 oz ground turkey

- 1 oz chives, chopped

- 1 teaspoon salt

- 1 teaspoon dried cilantro

- 1 teaspoon olive oil

- 1 teaspoon dried dill

- 1 egg white

- ¼ cup of water

Directions:

1. Put the ground turkey and chives in the mixing bowl.
2. Add salt, dried cilantro, dried dill, and egg white.
3. Stir the mixture until it is homogenous.
4. Brush the baking tray with olive oil.

5. Make the meatballs from the turkey mixture and put in the prepared baking tray. Add water.
6. Bake the meatballs for 25 minutes.

Nutrition value/serving:

calories 119, fat 6.9, fiber 0.1, carbs 0.3, protein 16.1

Raspberry and Apple Fruit Leather

Prep time: 10 minutes

Cooking time: 45 minutes

Servings: 6

Ingredients:

- 1 cup raspberries

- ½ cup apple, chopped

Directions:

1. Preheat the oven to 345F.
2. Line the baking tray with baking paper.
3. After this, put the raspberries and apples in the blender and blend until you get a smooth mixture.
4. Pour it in the baking tray and flatten well.
5. Bake the mixture for 45 minutes or until it is dry.
6. Then cut it into strips and roll into rolls.

Nutrition value/serving:

calories 20, fat 0.2, fiber 1.8, carbs 5, protein 0.3

Baked Apple with Hazelnuts

Prep time: 15 minutes

Cooking time: 20 minutes

Servings: 8

Ingredients:

- 4 Granny Smith apples

- 4 teaspoons almond butter

- 2 tablespoons raw honey

- 2 oz hazelnuts, chopped

Directions:

1. Cut the apples into halves and remove seeds.
2. Then make the medium size holes in the apple halves and fill them with almond butter, raw honey, and hazelnuts.
3. Place the apples in the tray and bake for 20 minutes at 350F.

Nutrition value/serving:

calories 167, fat 9, fiber 4.2, carbs 22.4, protein 3.1

Chocolate Energy Balls

Prep time: 15 minutes

Cooking time: 0 minutes

Servings: 5

Ingredients:

- 4 dates, chopped

- 3 oz cashew, chopped

- 1 tablespoon cocoa powder

Directions:

1. Put the dates in the blender and blend until you get a smooth mixture.
2. Then add cashew and cocoa powder.
3. Blend mixture for 30 seconds more.
4. Then remove it from the blender and make 5 energy balls with the help of the fingertips.

Nutrition value/serving:

calories 119, fat 8.1, fiber 1.4, carbs 11.1, protein 3

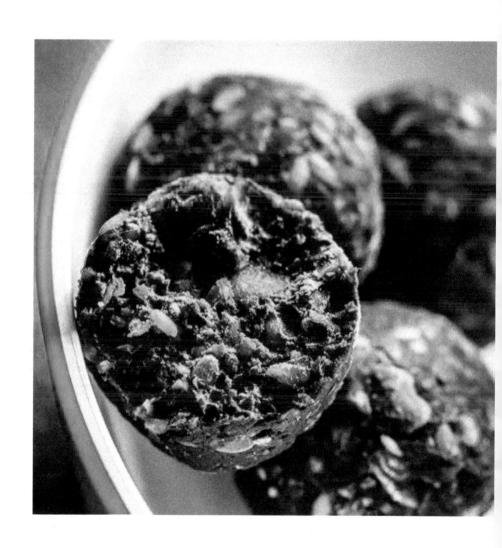

POULTRY

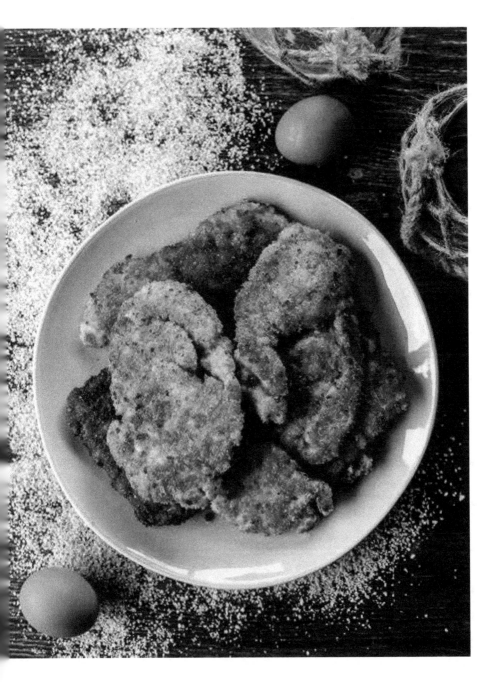

Chinese Chicken Salad

Prep time: 10 minutes

Cooking time: 10 minutes

Servings: 4

Ingredients:

- ½ cup purple cabbage, shredded

- 1 tablespoon chives, chopped

- 1 tablespoon almonds, chopped

- ½ red onion, chopped

- 1 teaspoon garlic powder

- 1 tablespoon sesame oil

- 8 oz chicken fillet, chopped

- ½ teaspoon salt

- 1 tangerine, chopped

- 1 teaspoon olive oil

Directions:

1. Heat up olive oil in the skillet.
2. Add chicken fillet.

3. Then sprinkle it with garlic powder and salt.

4. Roast the chicken for 10 minutes.

5. After this, transfer the cooked chicken in the big salad bowl.

6. Add shredded cabbage, chives, almonds, onion, sesame oil, and tangerine.

7. Shake the salad well.

Nutrition value/serving:

calories 167, fat 9.6, fiber 0.8, carbs 2.7, protein 17.1

Turmeric Chicken Soup

Prep time: 10 minutes

Cooking time: 30 minutes

Servings: 6

Ingredients:

- 4 cups chicken broth

- 6 chicken drumsticks

- 2 oz leek, chopped

- 1 tablespoon fresh dill, chopped

- 1 teaspoon ground turmeric

- 1 tablespoon coconut cream

- 1 teaspoon dried thyme

- 1 teaspoon salt

- 1 teaspoon olive oil

Directions:

1. Pour the olive oil in the saucepan and heat it up.
2. Add chicken drumsticks and roast them for 1 minute from each side on the high heat.

3. After this, add chicken broth, leek, dill, turmeric, thyme, and salt.

4. Bring the mixture to boil and add coconut cream.

5. Close the lid and simmer the soup on the medium heat for 20 minutes.

Nutrition value/serving:

calories 125, fat 5, fiber 0.4, carbs 2.7, protein 16.2

Shawarma Salad

Prep time: 10 minutes

Cooking time: 12 minutes

Servings: 4

Ingredients:

- 2 cups lettuce, chopped

- 1 red onion, sliced

- 1 cucumber, sliced

- 1 teaspoon tahini paste

- 1 teaspoon lemon juice

- 2 tablespoons water

- 1 teaspoon avocado oil

- 1 teaspoon salt

- 1 teaspoon ground black pepper

- 1 teaspoon Shawarma seasonings

- 8 oz chicken fillet

- 1 teaspoon sesame oil

Directions:

1. Rub the chicken with ground black pepper and salt.

2. Then brush it with avocado oil.

3. Preheat the grill to 375F.

4. Put the chicken in the grill and cook it for 6 minutes from each side.

5. Meanwhile, in the mixing bowl mix up lettuce, onion, and cucumber.

6. In the shallow bowl make the dressing: whisk together tahini paste, lemon juice, water, and sesame oil.

7. Chop the cooked chicken roughly and put over the salad mixture.

8. Then sprinkle the salad with Shawarma seasonings and top with dressing.

9. Give a good shake to the salad before serving.

Nutrition value/serving:

calories 154, fat 6.3, fiber 1.5, carbs 6.8, protein 17.6

Crusted Chicken Cutlets

Prep time: 10 minutes

Cooking time: 10 minutes

Servings: 2

Ingredients:

- 8 oz chicken fillet

- 2 eggs, beaten

- ½ cup almond flour

- ½ teaspoon salt

- ½ teaspoon ground black pepper

- 1 tablespoon avocado oil

Directions:

1. Cut the chicken fillet on 2 servings and beat them gently with the help of the kitchen hammer.
2. Then rub the chicken with salt and ground black pepper.
3. Heat up avocado oil in the skillet.
4. Then dip the chicken cutlets in the egg and coat in the almond flour. Repeat the same steps again.

5. After this, transfer the chicken cutlets in the hot oil and cook for 10 minutes. Flip the chicken on another side from time to time to avoid burning.

Nutrition value/serving:

calories 329, fat 17.2, fiber 1.2, carbs 2.6, protein 40

Huli Huli Chicken

Prep time: 20 minutes

Cooking time: 20 minutes

Servings: 2

Ingredients:

- 1 teaspoon pineapple juice

- 2 chicken thighs, skinless, boneless

- 1 teaspoon coconut aminos

- 1 teaspoon raw honey

- 1 teaspoon chives, chopped

- 1 teaspoon minced garlic

- 1 teaspoon ginger paste

- 1 teaspoon pineapple, chopped

- 1 teaspoon avocado oil

Directions:

1. Put the chicken thighs in the bowl and sprinkle them with coconut aminos, pineapple juice, raw honey, chives, minced garlic, ginger paste, and avocado oil.

2. Mix up the chicken thighs well and leave for 20 minutes to marinate.
3. After this, heat up the skillet well and arrange the chicken thighs inside.
4. Cook them for 10 minutes on the medium heat and then flip on another side.
5. Cook the chicken thighs for 10 minutes more.
6. After this, transfer the chicken in the plates and top with pineapple.

Nutrition value/serving:

calories 154, fat 7.4, fiber 0.3, carbs 5.2, protein 19.3

Shredded Pesto Chicken

Prep time: 15 minutes

Cooking time: 45 minutes

Servings: 4

Ingredients:

- 1-pound chicken breast, skinless, boneless

- 2 tablespoons pesto sauce (paleo)

- 1 bay leaf

- 1 teaspoon peppercorns

- 1 cup of water

Directions:

1. Pour water in the saucepan.
2. Add chicken breast, bay leaf, and peppercorns.
3. Close the lid and simmer the chicken for 45 minutes.
4. Then remove it from the water and shred with the help of the fork.
5. Add 2 tablespoons of the hot liquid from saucepan.
6. Then add pesto sauce and stir well.

Nutrition value/serving:

calories 165, fat 6.1, fiber 0.3, carbs 1, protein 24.9

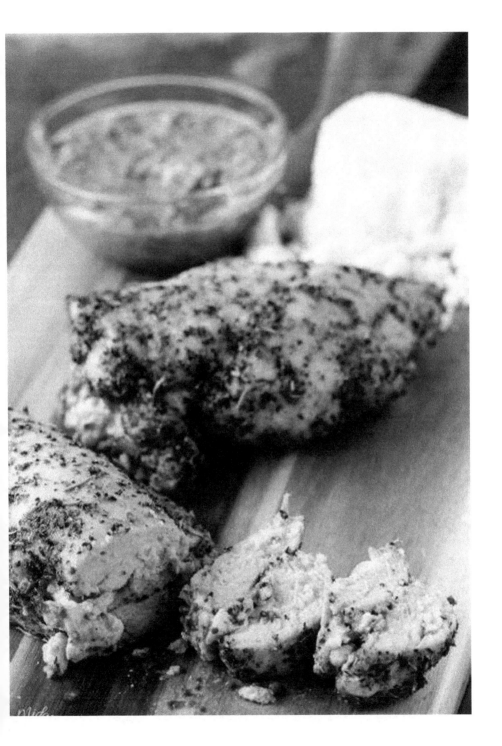

MEAT

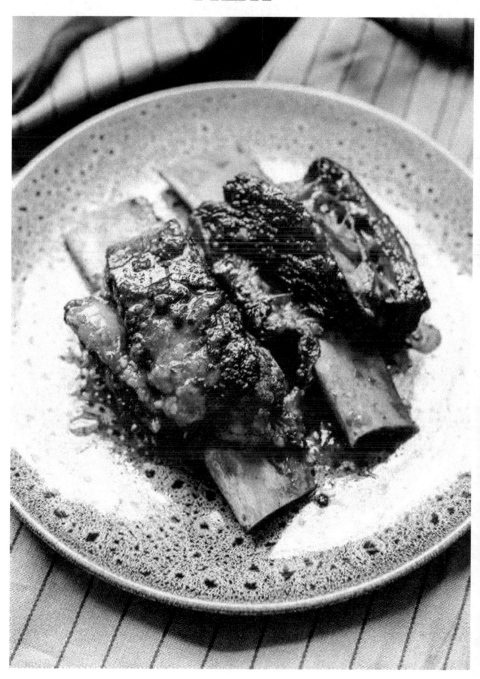

Beef Liver with Onion Gravy

Prep time: 15 minutes

Cooking time: 45 minutes

Servings: 4

Ingredients:

- 1-pound beef liver

- 1 onion, diced

- 1 teaspoon salt

- 1 tablespoon apple cider vinegar

- 2 cups of water

- 1 bay leaf

- 1 teaspoon chili flakes

- 1 tablespoon sesame oil

- 1 teaspoon coconut oil

- 1 teaspoon minced garlic

- ½ cup chicken stock

Directions:

1. Pour water in the saucepan and add the bay leaf.
2. Then add the beef liver and close the lid.
3. Boil it for 25 minutes.
4. After this, remove the beef liver from the saucepan and slice into servings.
5. Melt the coconut oil in the skillet.
6. Add minced garlic, chili flakes, salt, and diced onion.
7. Cook the ingredients until they are soft.
8. Then add sliced beef liver, apple cider vinegar, sesame oil, and chicken stock.
9. Close the lid and simmer the meal for 10 minutes on the medium-low heat.

Nutrition value/serving:

calories 253, fat 10, fiber 0.7, carbs 9, protein 30.5

Stuffed Peppers

Prep time: 20 minutes

Cooking time: 30 minutes

Servings: 4

Ingredients:

- 4 bell peppers, trimmed

- 1 cup ground beef

- ½ cup ground pork

- 1 teaspoon minced garlic

- 1 jalapeno pepper, minced

- 1 teaspoon salt

- ½ cup carrot, grated

- 1 cup beef broth

- 1 tablespoon avocado oil

Directions:

1. Remove the seeds from the bell peppers.
2. After this, in the mixing bowl mix up ground beef, ground pork, minced garlic, minced jalapeno, salt, and grated carrot.
3. Then fill the bell peppers with the ground meat mixture.

4. Brush the casserole mold with avocado oil and put the bell peppers inside.

5. Add beef broth and cover the mold with foil. Secure the edges of the mold.

6. Preheat the oven to 365F.

7. Put the mold with stuffed peppers in the oven and cook them for 30 minutes.

Nutrition value/serving:

calories 184, fat 6.7, fiber 2.2, carbs 11.2, protein 20.1

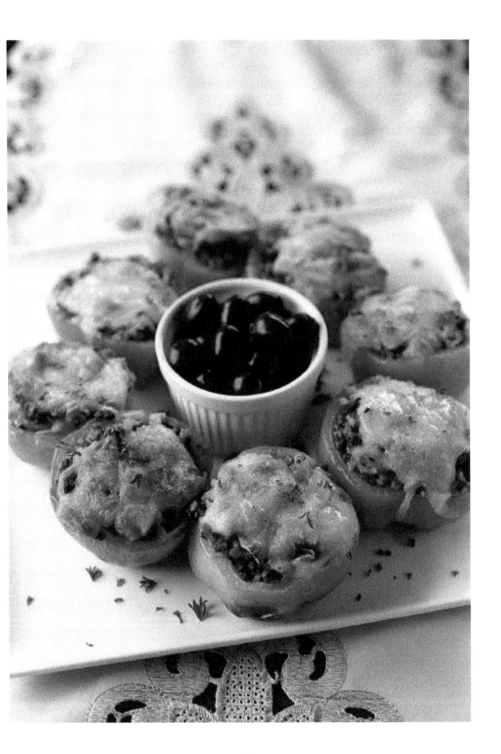

Hamburger Salad

Prep time: 15 minutes

Cooking time: 10 minutes

Servings: 5

Ingredients:

- 2 cups lettuce

- 1 cup ground beef

- 1 tablespoon minced onion

- 1 red onion, sliced

- 1 cup cherry tomatoes, halved

- ½ cup green olives, chopped

- 1 tablespoon sesame oil

- 1 teaspoon salt

- 1 tablespoon avocado oil

- ½ teaspoon chili flakes

- 1 tablespoon lemon juice

Directions:

1. In the mixing bowl mix up ground beef, minced onion, salt, and chili flakes.
2. Then make the mini burgers from the meat mixture.
3. Heat up avocado oil in the skillet and put the burgers inside.
4. Roast them for 4 minutes from each side.
5. Meanwhile, in the salad bowl mix up sliced onion, cherry tomatoes, green olives, sesame oil, and lemon juice.
6. Add the cooked mini burgers and shake the salad well.

Nutrition value/serving:

calories 103, fat 7.5, fiber 1.1, carbs 3.3, protein 5.9

Korean Style Pork Ribs

Prep time: 20 minutes

Cooking time: 25 minutes

Servings: 4

Ingredients:

- 16 oz pork spare ribs, chopped

- ½ apple, chopped

- 4 tablespoons coconut aminos

- 1 teaspoon sesame seeds

- 1 tablespoon sesame oil

- 1 tablespoon scallions, chopped

- 1 garlic clove, diced

Directions:

1. In the mixing bowl, mix up coconut aminos, sesame seeds, sesame oil, scallions, and diced garlic.
2. Then sprinkle the ribs with the sesame mixture and leave for 15-20 minutes to marinate.
3. Heat up the skillet well.

4. Put the spare ribs in the hot skillet and cook them for 7 minutes from each side on the medium heat.
5. Then sprinkle the ribs with remaining sesame mixture and add chopped apples.
6. Close the lid and cook the meal on low heat for 10 minutes.

Nutrition value/serving:

calories 278, fat 18, fiber 0.8, carbs 7.4, protein 20.5

Beef Pot Roast

Prep time: 10 minutes

Cooking time: 75 minutes

Servings: 6

Ingredients:

- 1 tablespoon fresh thyme

- 1 tablespoon fresh rosemary

- 2 carrots, roughly chopped

- 2 cups of water

- 1-pound beef chuck roast, roughly chopped

- 1 teaspoon salt

- 1 teaspoon ground black pepper

- 2 pears, chopped

- 1 tablespoon coconut oil

Directions:

1. Grease the pot with coconut oil.
2. Then put the chopped carrots, beef, and pears in the prepared pot.

3. Add ground black pepper, salt, water, rosemary, and thyme.
4. Preheat the oven to 365F.
5. Put the pot with ingredients in the preheated oven and cook it for 75 minutes.

Nutrition value/serving:

calories 347, fat 23.5, fiber 3.2, carbs 13.5, protein 20.3

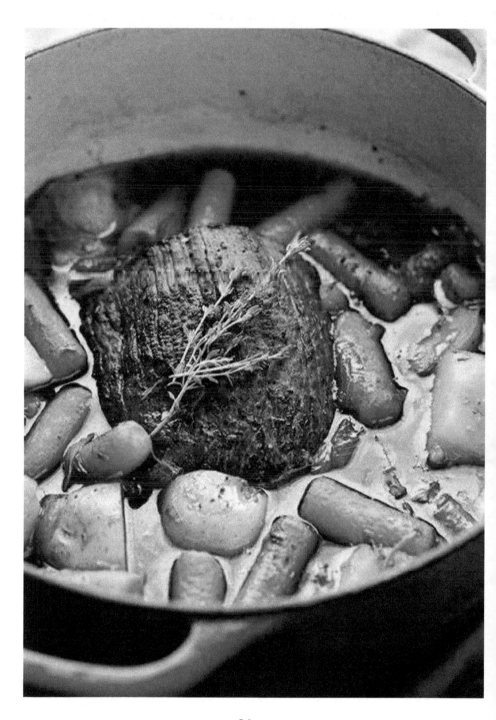

Marinated Bison Sirloin

Prep time: 40 minutes

Cooking time: 7 minutes

Servings: 4

Ingredients:

- 14 oz bison sirloin

- 2 tablespoons apple cider vinegar

- ½ orange

- 1 teaspoon ground nutmeg

- 1 teaspoon salt

- 2 tablespoons coconut aminos

- 1 teaspoon flax meal

- 1 teaspoon coconut flour

- 1 teaspoon cayenne pepper

- 2 tablespoons avocado oil

Directions:

1. In the mixing bowl, mix up bison sirloin, apple cider vinegar, ground nutmeg, salt, coconut aminos, cayenne pepper, and avocado oil.
2. Then squeeze the orange over the meat and shake it well.
3. Leave the meat in the marinade for 30 minutes.
4. Then preheat the grill to 390F.
5. Slice the meat and coat it in the mixture of flax meal and coconut flour.
6. Put the meat in the hot grill and cook it for 7 minutes.

Nutrition value/serving:

calories 209, fat 7.1, fiber 1.5, carbs 5.7, protein 28.5

FISH

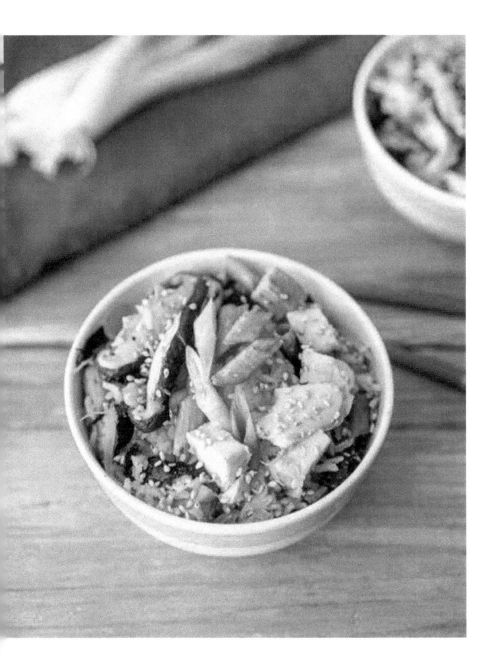

Shrimps and Chicken Skewers

Prep time: 20 minutes

Cooking time: 12 minutes

Servings: 4

Ingredients:

- 14 oz chicken fillet

- 14 oz shrimps, peeled

- 1 tablespoon lemon juice

- 1 teaspoon tomato paste

- 2 tablespoons sesame oil

- 1 teaspoon dried cilantro

- ½ teaspoon salt

Directions:

1. Chop the chicken fillet roughly.
2. In the mixing bowl mix up chopped chicken, shrimps, lemon juice, tomato paste, sesame oil, dried cilantro, and salt.
3. Then string the meat on the skewers and put in the preheated to 375F grill.
4. Cook the meal for 6 minutes from each side.

Nutrition value/serving:

calories 369, fat 15.9, fiber 0.1, carbs 1.8, protein 51.4

Sushi Bowl

Prep time: 10 minutes

Cooking time: 10 minutes

Servings: 2

Ingredients:

- 1 cup cauliflower, shredded

- 1 tablespoon olive oil

- ½ teaspoon salt

- ¼ cup of water

- 2 cucumbers, chopped

- 2 carrots, peeled, chopped

- 10 oz smoked salmon, sliced

- 2 oz seaweed

- ½ avocado, sliced

- 2 tablespoons coconut aminos

- 1 teaspoon sesame seeds

Directions:

1. Pour olive oil in the skillet and preheat it well.
2. Then add shredded cauliflower and sprinkle it with salt.
3. Add water and close the lid.
4. Cook the cauliflower for 7 minutes on the medium heat. Stir it from time to time.
5. Then transfer the cooked cauliflower in the serving bowls.
6. Top the cauliflower with smoked salmon, sliced avocado, cucumber, and carrot.
7. Sprinkle sushi bowls with sesame seeds, coconut aminos, and add the seaweed.

Nutrition value/serving:

calories 298, fat 16.1, fiber 5.4, carbs 20, protein 20.7

Cod Patties with Chives

Prep time: 20 minutes

Cooking time: 25 minutes

Servings: 4

Ingredients:

- 1-pound cod fillet

- 1 teaspoon ground coriander

- 1 tablespoon coconut oil

- 1 teaspoon minced garlic

- 1 tablespoon chives, chopped

- 2 tablespoons coconut flour

- ¼ cup of water

- ½ teaspoon salt

Directions:

1. Grind the cod fillet and mix it up with ground coriander, minced garlic, chives, coconut flour, and salt.
2. Make the medium size patties from the fish mixture.
3. Grease the baking pan with coconut oil.

4. Arrange the fish patties in the prepared baking pan.

5. Add water and transfer it in the preheated to 365F oven.

6. Bake the patties for 25 minutes.

Nutrition value/serving:

calories 139, fat 5.1, fiber 1.5, carbs 2.5, protein 21.1

Tuna Salad Verrine

Prep time: 15 minutes

Cooking time: 0 minutes

Servings: 6

Ingredients:

- 1-pound tuna, cooked

- 2 oz celery stalk, chopped

- 1 oz green onion, chopped

- ½ cup cucumbers, chopped

- 1 cup tomato, chopped

- ½ cup sweet pepper, chopped

- 2 tablespoons coconut cream

- 1 tablespoon lemon juice

- ½ teaspoon chili flakes

- 1 teaspoon dried oregano

Directions:

1. Chop the tuna roughly and put it in the salad bowl.

2. Add celery stalk, green onion, cucumbers, tomato, sweet pepper, and dried oregano. Mix up the salad.
3. After this, in the mixing bowl mix up chili flakes, lemon juice, and coconut cream. The dressing is cooked.
4. Sprinkle the salad with the dressing and shake gently.

Nutrition value/serving:

calories 166, fat 7.5, fiber 1, carbs 3.4, protein 20.8

Salmon Poke Bowl

Prep time: 10 minutes

Cooking time: 5 minutes

Servings: 2

Ingredients:

- 1 cup cauliflower, shredded

- 1 tablespoon lemon juice

- ¼ teaspoon salt

- ¼ teaspoon coconut sugar

- 1 oz pickled ginger, sliced

- 8 oz wild-caught salmon

- 1 teaspoon sesame seeds

- 2 tablespoons coconut aminos

- 1 teaspoon lime juice

- 1 cup of water

Directions:

1. Bring the water to boil and add shredded cauliflower.
2. Boil the vegetables for 3 minutes and then remove from water.

3. Add lemon juice, salt, and coconut sugar.
4. Stir the cauliflower well and transfer in the serving bowls.
5. After this, chop the salmon and mix it up with coconut aminos and lime juice.
6. Add the salmon in the cauliflower.
7. Then add sliced pickled ginger.
8. Sprinkle the meal with sesame seeds.

Nutrition value/serving:

calories 296, fat 10.9, fiber 3.3, carbs 17, protein 31.5

Smoked Salmon with Avocado Mousse

Prep time: 10 minutes

Cooking time: 0 minutes

Servings: 4

Ingredients:

- 1 avocado, pitted, peeled

- ¼ teaspoon minced garlic

- 10 oz smoked salmon, sliced

- 1 tablespoon fresh dill, chopped

- 4 teaspoons coconut milk

- ¼ teaspoon cayenne pepper

Directions:

1. Chop the avocado roughly and put it in the blender.
2. Add minced garlic, coconut milk, and cayenne pepper.
3. Blend the avocado until you get a smooth mixture. Avocado mousse is cooked.
4. After this, transfer the avocado mousse in the small glasses.
5. Top every mousse glass with sliced salmon and fresh dill.

Nutrition value/serving:

calories 200, fat 14.1, fiber 3.6, carbs 5.2, protein 14.2

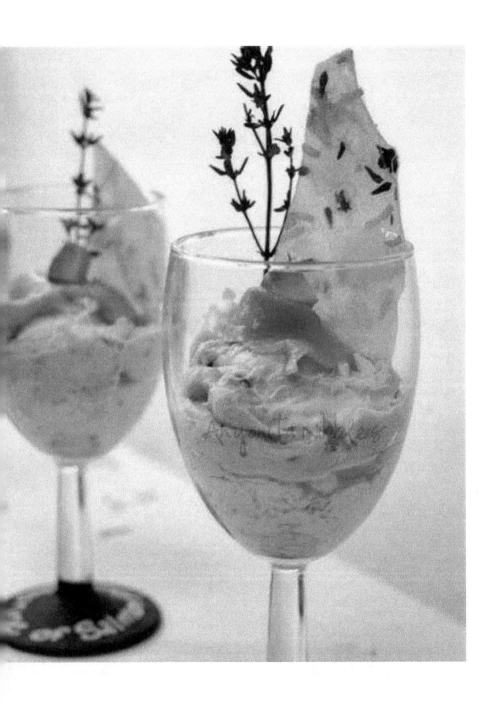

DESSERT

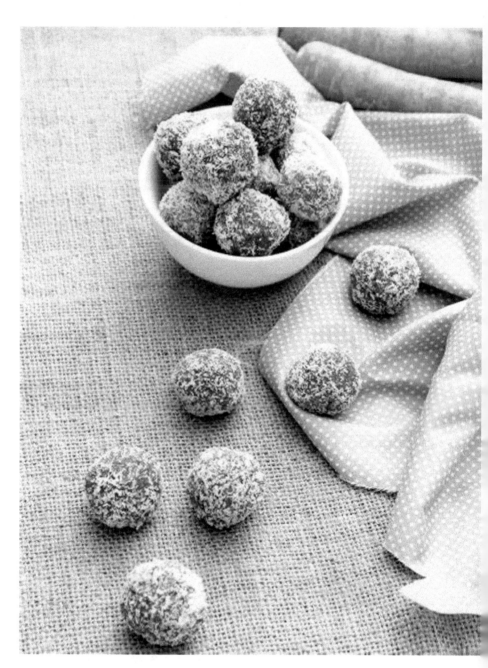

Peach Jam

Prep time: 10 minutes

Cooking time: 10 minutes

Servings: 4

Ingredients:

- 2 cups peaches, chopped

- 1 teaspoon ground cinnamon

- 1 anise star

- 1 tablespoon coconut sugar

Directions:

1. In the saucepan mix up peaches, ground cinnamon, and coconut sugar.
2. Add anise star.
3. Cook the mixture on the medium heat until coconut sugar is dissolved.
4. Then stir the lam mixture well and simmer it for 5 minutes.
5. Transfer the cooked jam in the glass jar and store it with the closed lid in the fridge.

Nutrition value/serving:
calories 50, fat 0.2, fiber 1.7, carbs 12, protein 1

Banana Pudding

Prep time: 15 minutes

Cooking time: 10 minutes

Servings: 4

Ingredients:

- 4 bananas, peeled, chopped

- 1 cup coconut cream

- 3 eggs yolk

- 1 teaspoon vanilla extract

Directions:

1. Smash the bananas and mix them up with coconut cream and vanilla extract.
2. Then add egg yolks and blend the mixture with the help of the immersion blender.
3. After this, transfer the smooth mixture on the heat and bring it to boil.
4. Simmer the pudding for 10 seconds and remove from the heat.
5. Transfer the cooked pudding into the serving bowls and cool well.

Nutrition value/serving:

calories 286, fat 18.1, fiber 4.4, carbs 30.9, protein 4.7

Lemon Bars

Prep time: 10 minutes

Cooking time: 20 minutes

Servings: 4

Ingredients:

- 1 cup tapioca flour

- 1 tablespoon raw honey

- 1 egg, beaten

- 1 teaspoon lemon zest

- ¼ cup lemon juice, freshly squeezed

- 1 teaspoon orange zest, grated

- 1 tablespoon cassava flour

- 1 egg yolk

- 1 teaspoon coconut flour

Directions:

1. In the mixing bowl mix up tapioca flour, raw honey, egg, lemon zest, lemon juice, orange zest, cassava flour, and coconut flour.

2. When the mixture is smooth, transfer it in the lined baking tray and flatten.
3. Bake the mixture for 20 minutes at 350F.
4. Then cut it on the bars and transfer in the serving plates.

Nutrition value/serving:

calories 173, fat 2.9, fiber 1.7, carbs 35.1, protein 2.8

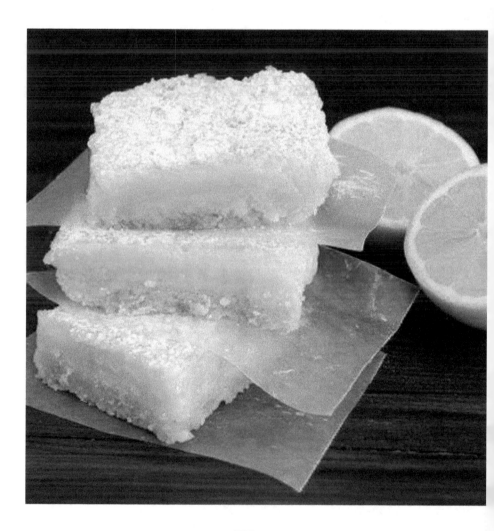

Fruit Sorbet

Prep time: 8 minutes

Cooking time: 0 minutes

Servings: 2

Ingredients:

- 1 banana, frozen, chopped

- 1/3 cup mango, chopped

- ½ cup organic almond milk

Directions:

1. Put the frozen banana, mango, and almond milk in the blender.
2. Blend the ingredients well and transfer them in the serving glasses.
3. Add ice cubes, if desired.

Nutrition value/serving:

calories 207, fat 14.6, fiber 3.3, carbs 20.9, protein 2.2

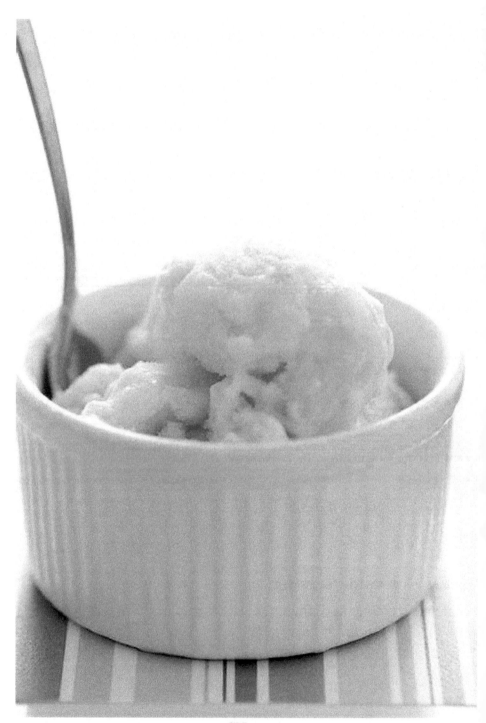

Carrot Energy Balls with Coconut

Prep time: 10 minutes

Cooking time: 0 minutes

Servings: 4

Ingredients:
- 2 carrots, peeled, grated
- 4 teaspoons coconut shred
- 4 pecans, chopped
- 4 tablespoons coconut flour
- 4 teaspoons honey
- 1 tablespoon almond flour

Directions:
1. Put the grated carrot in the bowl.
2. Add chopped pecans, coconut flour, almond flour, and honey.
3. Stir the mixture until smooth with the help of the fork.
4. Then make the small balls from the mixture and coat them in the coconut shred.

Nutrition value/serving:
calories 216, fat 15.4, fiber 6.1, carbs 17.7, protein 4.8

Strawberry Ice Cream

Prep time: 1 hour

Cooking time: 10 minutes

Servings: 2

Ingredients:

- 1 cup strawberries

- 1 avocado, peeled, pitted

- 1 tablespoon raw honey

Directions:

1. Chop the avocado and blend it until smooth.
2. Then add strawberries and blend the mixture for 2 minutes.
3. After this, add raw honey and pulse it for 30 seconds.
4. Put the mixture in the plastic vessel and freeze it for 1 hour. Stir it every 10 minutes.

Nutrition value/serving:

calories 260, fat 19.8, fiber 8.2, carbs 22.8 protein 2.4

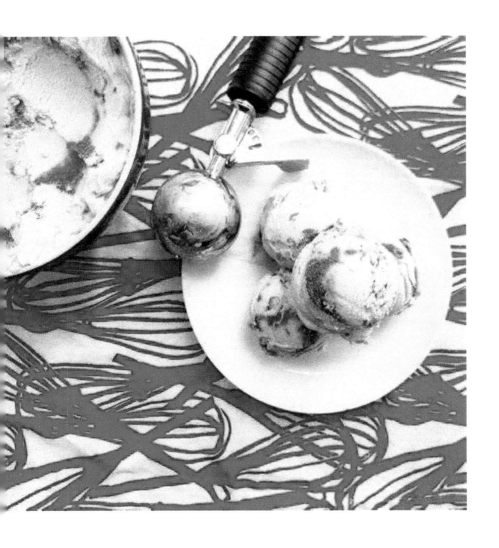

Lightning Source UK Ltd.
Milton Keynes UK
UKHW020923010721
386455UK00005B/50